THE KIDS CANCER COOKBOOK

Healthy and nutritious Cancer-Fighting Recipes for Kids

Autumn E. Clark

Copyright © 2023 Autumn E. Clark

Table of content

CHAPTER 8   42

Snack Options   42

CHAPTER 1

Introduction to Cancer and Nutrition

Cancer is a devastating and life-altering disease that affects millions of people around the world each year. While there are treatments available to help fight cancer, nutrition plays an important role in helping to prevent cancer as well as aiding in recovery for those who have been diagnosed.

Nutrition provides essential nutrients such as vitamins, minerals, proteins, and carbohydrates needed for healthy cell growth and development.

Proper nutrition can reduce the risk of developing certain types of cancers or slow down their progression if they do occur. It also helps to improve symptoms associated with cancer and its treatment, such as fatigue, nausea, pain, and loss of appetite.

The connection between diet and cancer has been explored extensively over the years by researchers studying both human populations and animal models.

This research has identified many dietary components that may influence cancer risk, including specific foods and food groups, supplements, and even the timing of meals.

It is important to note that while certain dietary components may have beneficial effects on cancer prevention or progression, there is still much to be learned about their exact role in this process.

Nutrition plays an important role in helping people maintain a healthy lifestyle, regardless of whether they are at risk for developing cancer or have already been diagnosed with it.

Eating a balanced diet full of fruits, vegetables, and whole grains can provide essential vitamins and minerals needed for proper cell growth and development as well as reduce inflammation throughout the body.

Dietary patterns such as plant-based eating can also help reduce the risk of chronic diseases, including cancer. Additionally, eating healthy foods and avoiding processed and high-fat foods can also help to control weight gain associated with certain cancer treatments.

In summary, nutrition plays an important role in both preventing and treating cancer. Eating a balanced diet full of fruits, vegetables, whole grains, and lean proteins can provide the nutrients needed for healthy cell growth and development as well as reduce inflammation throughout the body.

It is important to remember that while certain dietary components may have beneficial effects on reducing or slowing down cancer progression, further research is still needed to fully understand their exact role in this process

Understanding cancer and it's treatment

Cancer is a disease caused by the abnormal and uncontrolled growth of cells, which can form tumors or spread throughout the body. The term cancer encompasses many different types of diseases, all characterized by the development of abnormal cells that grow and divide without normal control mechanisms.

The exact cause of cancer is not known; however, environmental factors such as exposure to certain chemicals, radiation (including ultraviolet light), viruses, lifestyle choices (such as smoking), and genetic mutations are believed to contribute to its development. Not all cancers have a single cause—some may be due to multiple causes.

To diagnose cancer accurately, doctors use various tests including physical examinations, imaging scans (e.g., X-rays), laboratory tests (e.g., blood tests), and tissue biopsies. Once a diagnosis is made, the type of treatment will depend on the specific cancer and its stage (how far it has progressed).

Treatment options for cancer include surgery, radiation therapy, chemotherapy, and/or targeted therapies (such as monoclonal antibodies or immunotherapy). Surgery involves removing all or part of a tumor; radiation therapy uses high-energy X-rays to kill cancer cells; while chemotherapy and targeted therapies use drugs to destroy cancer cells. Other treatments may also be used depending on the individual case.

In addition to these treatments, supportive care is also essential in helping patients manage their symptoms and side effects during treatment. This can include pain relief medications, nutritional support, psychological counseling, and physical therapy.

Cancer is a complex and challenging disease, but with the right treatment plan, it can often be managed effectively. The key to successful treatment is early detection, so if you have any concerns or symptoms that could indicate cancer, it's important to discuss them with your doctor as soon as possible.

The importance of good nutrition during cancer treatment

Good nutrition is an essential part of cancer treatment and recovery and can help improve your overall well-being during this difficult time.

Eating a well-balanced diet full of nutrient-dense foods will provide the energy needed for healing; reduce side effects from chemotherapy, radiation therapy, or other treatments; protect cells from damage caused by treatments; and reduce the risk of developing certain types of cancers.

A healthy diet includes fruits, vegetables, whole grains, lean proteins (such as fish or poultry), low-fat dairy products, nuts, and seeds, legumes such as beans or lentils; and healthy fats like olive oil or avocado. It's important to limit processed foods that are high in sugar, unhealthy fats (including trans fats) saturated fat, and salt/sodium.

Eating a well-balanced diet may help improve your overall well-being and prevent weight loss, a common side effect of cancer treatment.

Eating foods rich in antioxidants may also help protect your cells from the damage caused by chemotherapy or radiation therapy. Additionally, some studies have suggested that a diet high in fruits and vegetables may reduce the risk of developing certain types of cancers.

During cancer treatment, you may need additional calories and nutrients to keep up with the body's increased need for energy and healing.

You should focus on eating nutrient-dense foods like lean proteins, whole grains, healthy fats (such as olive oil or avocado), dairy products low in fat, fresh fruits and vegetables; nuts; legumes such as beans or lentils; and omega-3 fatty acids found in fish and fish oil supplements.

It's also important to stay hydrated by drinking plenty of fluids, such as water, herbal teas, and fruit juices. Your doctor may recommend that you take a multivitamin or other dietary supplement to help ensure that you are getting enough vitamins and minerals.

You should talk to your doctor before taking any supplement, as some can interfere with medications or treatments for cancer. Be sure to talk with your doctor or a registered dietitian before making any changes to your diet during cancer treatment.

CHAPTER 2

The basics of a healthy diet

A healthy diet is one of the most important aspects of good nutrition for children. Eating a balanced and varied diet can help them to grow up strong and healthy while reducing their risk of developing many diseases, including cancer.

The basics of a healthy diet are simple: Eat plenty of fruits and vegetables, whole grains, lean proteins, low-fat dairy products, nuts and seeds, legumes (beans), fatty fish such as salmon or tuna at least twice per week, and limit processed foods with added sugar or sodium (salt).

Avoid unhealthy fats such as trans fats in margarine and fast food. Choose water instead of sugary drinks whenever possible.

1. Fruits and Vegetables: Fruits and vegetables should make up about half of a child's plate. Eating plenty of fruits and vegetables provides essential vitamins, minerals, fiber, and antioxidants that help protect against cancer and other diseases. Choose fresh or frozen fruits and vegetables whenever possible; canned varieties often contain added sodium or sugar.

2. Whole Grains: Whole grains are an important source of B vitamins, iron, zinc, magnesium, and dietary fiber which can help reduce the risk of certain types of cancer as well as other chronic diseases such as type 2 diabetes. Examples of whole grains include brown rice, quinoa, oats, barley, buckwheat, and bulgur wheat.

3. Proteins: Protein helps your child build strong muscles and bones while providing energy for growth. Lean proteins such as fish, poultry, and legumes (beans) are good sources of protein. Limit processed meats such as bacon and hot dogs which can be high in sodium and unhealthy fats.

4. Low-Fat Dairy Products: Low-fat dairy products provide calcium which is important for strong bones and teeth. Choose low-fat or fat-free milk, yogurt, cheese, or other dairy products made from skim milk or 2% milk instead of higher-fat versions.

5. Nuts & Seeds: Nuts and seeds contain healthy fats that can help reduce inflammation in the body while providing essential vitamins, minerals, fiber, and proteins. Examples include almonds, walnuts, sunflower seeds, and pumpkin seeds. Be sure to choose unsalted varieties whenever possible

6. Legumes (Beans): Legumes are a great source of protein, fiber, and other essential vitamins and minerals. Examples include lentils, kidney beans, black beans, chickpeas, and soybeans.

7. Fatty Fish: Eating fatty fish such as salmon or tuna at least twice per week can provide important omega-3 fatty acids that help reduce inflammation in the body which can protect against certain types of cancer.

8. Limit Processed Foods: Processed foods often contain added sugar or sodium (salt) that can be unhealthy for your child's diet. Choose whole grains over refined grains whenever possible; choose fresh fruits and vegetables instead of canned varieties; limit processed meats such as bacon and hot dogs; avoid sugary drinks and choose water instead.

These are the basics of a healthy diet for children that can help protect them against cancer and other chronic diseases. Eating a balanced and varied diet is an important part of good nutrition, so be sure to include these foods in your child's meals whenever possible.

CHAPTER 3

Shopping and meal planning tips

Shopping and meal planning for a cancer patient can be a daunting task. It is important to consider the nutritional needs of the individual when creating meals and snacks. The American Cancer Society (ACS) recommends that all individuals, including those with cancer, follow general nutrition guidelines from the Dietary Guidelines for Americans.

When shopping for food, it is important to choose nutrient-rich foods such as fruits, vegetables, whole grains, lean meats and fish, low-fat dairy products, beans, and legumes. These foods are high in vitamins and minerals while also being low in calories which can help maintain a healthy weight during treatment.

It is also important to limit processed foods such as refined carbohydrates like white bread or pasta; sugary drinks like sodas; and fried foods.

Meal preparation is greatly facilitated by meal planning, which is also a fantastic way to make sure that cancer patients are getting the nutrition they require. Start by planning your meals for the entire week, including breakfast, lunch, dinner, and snacks. Include a lot of fruits, vegetables, and lean proteins, such as chicken or fish. For extra taste and texture, use small amounts of healthy fats like nuts, seeds, avocados, or olive oil.

To avoid being bored with the same foods every week, try to include variety in your meals. Throughout the day, it's crucial to stay hydrated by drinking lots of water or other calorie-free liquids like herbal teas or sparkling water with lemon juice.

When preparing meals, choose cooking methods like baking, roasting, or grilling instead of frying. Consider using herbs and spices to add flavor rather than salt.

It is also important to pay attention to portion sizes and be mindful of how much you are eating. Eating smaller portions more often can help with nausea that is common during treatment.

You can make sure your loved one with cancer gets the nutrients they require while still enjoying tasty meals by following this shopping and meal-planning advice based on cancer nutrition standards.

CHAPTER 4

Easy Recipes for cancer-fighting meals

Here are some easy recipes that incorporate cancer-fighting ingredients:

Roasted Vegetable Quinoa Bowl

Ingredients:
- 1 cup quinoa, rinsed
- 2 bell peppers, roughly chopped
- 1 onion, diced
- 1 head of broccoli, cut into florets
- 2 tablespoons olive oil

Instructions:
1. Preheat the oven to 400°F. Cover a baking sheet with parchment paper.

2. Place the quinoa in a medium saucepan and add 2 cups of water. Bring to a boil over high heat then reduce the heat to low and simmer for 15 minutes or until all of the liquid is absorbed by the quinoa. Set aside when done cooking.

3. In a large bowl, combine the bell peppers, onion, and broccoli. Sprinkle with salt and pepper and drizzle with olive oil. Throw to cover in the oil and seasoning.

4. Spread the vegetables out onto the parchment-lined baking sheet in a single layer then roast for 20 minutes or until tender.

5. When ready to serve, divide quinoa between four bowls then top each one with roasted vegetables. Enjoy!

Lentil and Kale Stew

Ingredients:
- 1 tablespoon olive oil
- 1 onion, diced
- 2 cloves garlic, minced
- 2 carrots, chopped into small pieces
- 4 cups vegetable broth
- 1 cup dried green lentils, rinsed
- ½ teaspoon dried thyme leaves

Instructions:
1. Heat the olive oil in a big pot over medium intensity. Add the onions and garlic then sauté for 3 minutes or until softened.

2. Stir in the carrots then pour in the vegetable broth and lentils. Bring to a boil then reduce heat to low and simmer for 25 minutes or until lentils are tender.

3. Add the kale and thyme then cook for an additional 5 minutes or until the kale is wilted.

4. Serve warm with crusty bread or overcooked grains such as quinoa or rice. Enjoy!

Sweet Potato Curry

Ingredients:
- 2 tablespoons olive oil
- 1 onion, diced
- 2 cloves garlic, minced
- 1 tablespoon curry powder
- ¼ teaspoon cumin powder
- ½ teaspoon ground ginger
- 2 sweet potatoes, peeled and cubed into small pieces

Instructions:
1. Heat the olive oil in a big pot over medium intensity.Add the onions and garlic then sauté for 3 minutes or until softened.

2. Stir in the curry powder, cumin and ginger then cook for an additional minute to toast the spices.

3. Add the sweet potatoes then pour in 1 cup of water or vegetable broth. Bring to a boil then reduce the heat to low and simmer for 15 minutes or until potatoes are tender.

4. Serve over cooked grains such as quinoa or rice, with fresh cilantro on top if desired. Enjoy!

Spinach and Chickpea Salad

Ingredients:
- 2 cups spinach, washed and dried
- 1 can chickpeas (15 ounces), washed and rinsed
- ½ cup cherry tomatoes, halved - ¼ cup red onion, diced

Instructions:
1. In a large bowl combine the spinach, chickpeas, tomatoes, and onions then toss together until evenly mixed.

2.Sprinkle with salt and pepper and drizzle with olive oil.. Coat the items in oil and seasoning by tossing them.

3. Serve as is or topped with a drizzle of balsamic vinegar or lemon juice, if desired. Enjoy!

Mediterranean Baked Fish with Tomatoes, Olives, and Feta Cheese

Ingredients:
- 2 tablespoons olive oil
- 1 tablespoon lemon juice
- 1 teaspoon dried oregano
- 4 (4 ounce) white fish fillets such as cod or halibut

- ½ cup cherry tomatoes, halved
- ¼ cup kalamata olives, pitted and sliced 2 tablespoons crumbled feta cheese

Instructions:

1. Preheat oven to 400°F. Cover a baking sheet with parchment paper.

2. In a small bowl combine the olive oil, lemon juice, and oregano then whisk together until mixed.

3. Place the fish fillets on the parchment-lined baking sheet then brush each one generously with the olive oil mixture.

4. Top each fillet with tomatoes, olives, and feta cheese then bake for 15 minutes or until fish is cooked through and flakes easily when tested with a fork.

5. Serve warm over cooked grains such as quinoa or rice if desired Enjoy!

Grilled Salmon with Asparagus and Lemon-Garlic Sauce

Ingredients:
- 2 tablespoons olive oil
- 1 tablespoon lemon juice

- 1 teaspoon minced garlic - 4 (4 ounce) salmon fillets Salt and pepper, to taste

Instructions:
1. Set a grill or grill pan to medium-high heat and allow it to preheat. Brush lightly with oil if needed.

2. In a small bowl combine the olive oil, lemon juice, and garlic then whisk together until mixed.

3. Season both sides of the salmon fillets generously with salt and pepper then place on the preheated grill or grill pan skin side up (if applicable). Cook for 5 minutes without moving then flip and cook for an additional 5 minutes or until cooked through.

4. When ready to serve, brush each fillet with the lemon-garlic sauce and top with grilled asparagus if desired. Enjoy!

Brown Rice Bowl with Edamame, Mushrooms, Zucchini, Peppers, and Onions

Ingredients:
- 2 tablespoons olive oil
- 1 cup brown rice
- 2 cups vegetable broth
- ½ cup edamame beans, shelled and cooked according to package instructions Salt and pepper, to taste

Instructions:
1. Heat the olive oil in a big pot over medium intensity. Add the onions and garlic then sauté for 3 minutes or until softened.

2. Stir in the brown rice then pour in the vegetable broth. Bring to a boil then reduce heat to low and simmer for 25 minutes or until all of the liquid is absorbed by the rice.

3. When the rice is almost done cooking, add in the edamame beans and vegetables then season with salt and pepper. Boil vegetables for an extra 5 minutes or until they are soft.

4. Serve warm as is or topped with grilled salmon if desired Enjoy!

Garlic Shrimp Stir Fry with Broccoli Rabe

Ingredients:
- 2 tablespoons olive oil
- 1 pound shrimp, peeled and deveined
- 2 cloves garlic, minced
- 1 bunch broccoli rabe, trimmed and cut into pieces Salt and pepper, to taste

Instructions:

1. Heat the olive oil in a huge skillet over medium intensity. Add the shrimp then season with salt and pepper. Cook for 3 minutes or until just starting to turn pink then add the garlic and cook for an additional minute.

2. Add in the broccoli rabe then stir fry together for 5 minutes or until the shrimp is cooked through and the vegetables are tender.

3. Serve warm over cooked grains such as quinoa or rice, with fresh lemon wedges if desired. Enjoy!

Curried Red Lentil Soup

Ingredients:
- 2 tablespoons olive oil
- 1 onion, diced
- 2 cloves garlic, minced
- 1 tablespoon curry powder
- ½ teaspoon cumin powder
- ¼ teaspoon ground ginger
- 1 cup red lentils, rinsed
- 4 cups vegetable broth

Instructions:

1. Heat the olive oil in a big pot over medium intensity. Add the onions and garlic then sauté for 3 minutes or until softened.

2. Stir in the curry powder, cumin and ginger then cook for an additional minute to toast the spices.

3. Pour in the lentils and vegetable broth then bring to a boil before reducing the heat to low and simmering for 20 minutes or until lentils are tender.

4. Serve warm as is or topped with fresh chopped parsley if desired Enjoy!

Avocado & Black Bean Burrito Bowls

Ingredients:
- 2 tablespoons olive oil
-1 onion, diced
- 2 cloves garlic, minced
- 1 teaspoon ground cumin
- ½ teaspoon chili powder
- 1 can black beans (15 ounces), drained and rinsed Salt and pepper, to taste

Instructions:
1. Heat the olive oil in a huge skillet over medium intensity. Add the onions and garlic then sauté for 3 minutes or until softened.
2. Stir in the cumin and chili powder then cook for an additional minute to toast the spices.

3. Add in the black beans then season with salt and pepper if desired before cooking for an additional 5 minutes or until heated through.

4. Serve warm over cooked grains such as quinoa or rice, with fresh avocado and cilantro on top if desired. Enjoy!

CHAPTER 5

Breakfast Ideas

Overnight Oats with Berries and Chia Seeds

Mix 1/2 cup rolled oats, 1/2 cup milk or almond milk, 1/2 cup mixed berries, 1 tbsp chia seeds, and 1 tsp honey. Cover and refrigerate overnight. In the morning, top with more berries and a drizzle of honey.

Spinach and Mushroom Frittata

Whisk together 4 eggs, 1/2 cup chopped spinach, 1/2 cup chopped mushrooms, 1/4 cup grated cheese, and a pinch of salt. Pour the mixture into a greased muffin tin and bake at 350F for 20-25 minutes, or until the frittatas are set.

Avocado Toast with Egg

Mash 1/2 an avocado onto a piece of whole grain toast. Top with a fried or poached egg and sprinkle with a pinch of salt and pepper.

Banana and Peanut Butter Smoothie

Blend 1 banana, 1 cup unsweetened almond milk, 1 tbsp peanut butter, and a handful of ice. If preferred, incorporate a scoop of protein powder.

Sweet Potato and Egg Breakfast Hash

Dice 1 sweet potato and cook in a pan with a little oil over medium heat until tender. Break 2 eggs into the pan and cook until the whites become solid. Serve with some chopped fresh herbs on top.

Green Smoothie

Blend 1 cup spinach, 1 banana, 1/2 cup unsweetened almond milk, 1/2 cup frozen berries, and 1 tsp honey. If preferred, incorporate a scoop of protein powder.

Whole Grain Pancakes with Blueberries

In a bowl, whisk together 1 cup whole grain flour, 1 tsp baking powder, 1/2 tsp salt, and 1 cup milk or almond milk. Stir in 1/2 cup of blueberries. Cook spoonfuls of the batter in a greased pan over medium heat until bubbles form on the surface, then flip and cook until browned on both sides.

Mini Breakfast Burritos

Spread a whole grain tortilla with mashed avocado and scrambled eggs. Top with shredded cheese and a sprinkle of chopped herbs. Roll up the tortilla and slice it into small pieces.

Greek Yogurt Parfait

Layer Greek yogurt, mixed berries, and granola in a jar or cup. Top with a drizzle of honey.

Quinoa and Veggie Breakfast Bowl

Cook 1/2 cup quinoa according to package instructions. Top with roasted vegetables, a fried egg, and a sprinkle of feta cheese.

Whole Grain Waffles with Fresh Fruit

Make a batch of whole grain waffles according to the package instructions or your favorite recipe. Top with sliced fruit, such as bananas, berries, or peaches.

Chia Seed Pudding

Mix 1/4 cup chia seeds, 1 cup unsweetened almond milk, 1 tsp honey, and a pinch of cinnamon. Cover and refrigerate overnight. In the morning, top with sliced fruit and a sprinkle of nuts or shredded coconut.

Breakfast Tacos

Scramble eggs and fill small whole-grain tortillas with eggs, sliced avocado, diced tomato, and shredded cheese.

Apple and Almond Butter Sandwich

Spread almond butter on two slices of whole-grain bread. Top with cut apples and a shower of honey.

Tofu Scramble

Scramble firm tofu with diced vegetables, such as bell peppers, onions, and mushrooms. Season with turmeric, cumin, and paprika for a savory flavor. Serve on a whole-grain English muffin or in a whole-grain wrap.

CHAPTER 6

Lunch Options

Here are some lunch recipes that are packed with cancer-fighting nutrients:

Quinoa, black bean, and corn salad

Cook quinoa according to package instructions. In a separate pan, sauté black beans and corn in a little bit of oil until heated through. Mix the quinoa, black beans, and corn in a bowl and add some diced bell peppers and diced red onions. Dress with a mixture of lime juice, olive oil, cumin, and chili powder.

Peanut butter and banana wrap

Spread peanut butter and sliced bananas onto a whole wheat tortilla. Slice the tortilla into bite-sized pieces after rolling it up. Peanut butter is a good source of plant-based protein and bananas are high in potassium.

Turkey, hummus, and vegetable wrap

Spread hummus onto a whole wheat tortilla. Top with sliced turkey, diced bell peppers, and diced cucumbers. Slice the tortilla into bite-sized pieces after rolling it up. Hummus is made from chickpeas, which are high in fiber and protein, and the vegetables add a boost of vitamins and minerals.

Oven-baked sweet potato fries

Preheat the oven to 425°F. Cut sweet potatoes into thin fries and toss with a little bit of olive oil and your choice of seasonings (e.g. paprika, garlic powder, onion powder). Spread the fries onto a baking sheet in a single layer and bake for 20-25 minutes, or until crispy. Sweet potatoes are high in vitamin A, which can help boost the immune system.

Grilled chicken and vegetable skewers

Cut chicken breasts into small cubes and thread them onto skewers with your choice of vegetables (such as bell peppers, onions, and cherry tomatoes). Barbecue the skewers until the chicken is cooked through and the vegetables are delicate. Chicken is a good source of protein and vegetables add a boost of vitamins and minerals.

Roasted turkey and veggie quesadillas

Spread a layer of diced roasted turkey and your choice of vegetables (such as bell peppers, onions, and mushrooms) onto a whole wheat tortilla. Top with another tortilla and press delicately to seal. Heat a little bit of oil in a pan over medium heat and cook the quesadilla for 2-3 minutes on each side, or until the tortillas are crispy and the filling is hot.

Avocado and black bean salad

Mix mashed avocado, drained and rinsed black beans, diced cherry tomatoes, and diced red onion in a bowl. Squeeze a little bit of lime juice over the top and sprinkle with cumin and chili powder. Avocado is a good source of healthy fats and black beans are high in fiber and protein.

Greek yogurt with berries and nuts

Top a cup of Greek yogurt with a mixture of your favorite berries and a sprinkle of chopped nuts. Greek yogurt is high in protein and the berries and nuts add a boost of antioxidants and healthy fats.

Whole grain pasta with marinara sauce and vegetables

Cook whole grain pasta according to package instructions and toss with your favorite marinara sauce and a mixture of diced vegetables, such as bell peppers, onions, and zucchini. Whole grains are high in fiber, which can help protect against certain types of cancer.

Baked salmon with roasted vegetables

Preheat the oven to 400°F. Place a salmon fillet onto a baking sheet and top with your choice of vegetables (such as asparagus, cherry tomatoes, and bell peppers). Drizzle with a little bit of olive oil and sprinkle with your favorite seasonings. Bake for 10-12 minutes, or until the salmon is cooked through and the vegetables are tender. Salmon is a decent source of omega-3 unsaturated fats, which can assist with decreasing irritation in the body.

Black bean and corn salad with honey mustard dressing

In a bowl, mix canned black beans, frozen corn, diced bell peppers, and diced red onions. In a separate bowl, whisk together honey, mustard, apple cider vinegar, and a little bit of olive oil to make a dressing. Toss the black bean and corn mixture with the dressing to coat. Black beans and corn are high in fiber and the honey mustard dressing adds a touch of sweetness.

Whole grain pita with hummus and vegetables

Spread hummus onto a whole grain pita and top with your choices of sliced vegetables, such as cucumbers, bell peppers, and tomatoes. Whole grains are high in fiber, and vegetables and hummus add a boost of nutrients.

Turkey and cheese roll-ups

Spread a little bit of cream cheese onto a slice of deli turkey and roll up. Repeat with the remaining slices of turkey. The cream cheese adds a creamy texture and the turkey is a good source of protein.

Grilled chicken and fruit skewers

Thread diced grilled chicken onto skewers with your choice of fruit (such as pineapple, watermelon, and mango). The fruit adds a burst of sweetness and the chicken is a good source of protein.

Quinoa and black bean burrito bowls

Cook quinoa according to package instructions and mix with canned black beans, diced bell peppers, and diced red onions. Top with your favorite salsa and shredded cheese. Quinoa is a complete protein and black beans are high in fiber.

CHAPTER 7

Dinner Recipes

Here are some ideas for cancer-fighting dinner dishes for kids:

Grilled chicken with roasted vegetables

Grill some chicken breasts and serve with a side of roasted vegetables, like bell peppers, zucchini, and cherry tomatoes.

Turkey and black bean tacos

Top some whole grain tortillas with ground turkey, black beans, and a variety of vegetables, like lettuce, tomato, and avocado.

Whole grain spaghetti with turkey meatballs

Serve whole grain spaghetti with turkey meatballs and a side of steamed broccoli.

Salmon and sweet potato cakes

Bake or grill some salmon and serve with sweet potato cakes made from mashed sweet potatoes and whole grain flour.

Quinoa and black bean salad

Mix cooked quinoa with black beans, corn, cherry tomatoes, and avocado, and dress with a citrus vinaigrette.

Grilled tofu skewers with quinoa and roasted vegetables

Grill some tofu skewers and serve with a side of cooked quinoa and roasted vegetables, like asparagus and cherry tomatoes.

Baked chicken parmesan with whole grain spaghetti

Bake some chicken breasts coated in whole grain breadcrumbs and topped with tomato sauce and cheese, and serve with whole grain spaghetti.

Black bean and corn salad with grilled shrimp

Mix a salad of black beans, corn, cherry tomatoes, and avocado, and top with grilled shrimp.

Slow cooker lentil and vegetable soup

Put lentils, a variety of vegetables, and some broth in a slow cooker and let it cook until the lentils are tender.

Whole grain pizza with veggies and turkey sausage

Make a whole grain pizza crust and top it with tomato sauce, cheese, and a variety of vegetables, like bell peppers, onions, and mushrooms. Add some sliced turkey sausage for protein.

Grilled salmon with quinoa and steamed broccoli

Grill some salmon and serve with a side of cooked quinoa and steamed broccoli.

Baked turkey and vegetable empanadas

Mix some cooked ground turkey and a variety of vegetables, like bell peppers, onions, and corn, and put a spoonful of the mixture inside a whole-grain empanada wrapper. Bake until the wrapper is crispy.

Black bean and quinoa burgers with roasted sweet potatoes

Mix cooked black beans and quinoa, and form into patties. Grill or bake the patties and serve with roasted sweet potatoes.

Grilled chicken and vegetable kebabs with brown rice

Skewer some chicken breasts and a variety of vegetables, like bell peppers, onions, and cherry tomatoes, and grill until the chicken is cooked through. Brown rice should be served alongside.

Baked salmon with quinoa and steamed asparagus

Bake some salmon and serve with a side of cooked quinoa and steamed asparagus.

CHAPTER 8

Snack Options

Hummus and Veggie Wrap

Spread hummus on a whole wheat wrap, and layer with sliced cucumbers, tomatoes, and shredded carrots. Roll up the wrap and cut it into bite-sized pieces.

Yogurt Parfait

Layer low-fat vanilla yogurt with fresh berries and crushed graham crackers in a small cup or bowl.

Rice Cake Pizzas

Top brown rice cakes with tomato sauce, cheese, and favorite pizza toppings like mushrooms or olives for easy snacks kids will love!

Frozen Grapes

Place grapes onto a baking sheet lined with parchment paper; freeze until solid then store in an airtight container for a refreshing frozen treat!

Apple Sandwiches

Spread all-natural peanut butter on two slices of whole wheat bread and layer with thinly sliced apples.

Trail Mix

Combine unsalted nuts, dried fruit, and dark chocolate chips for tasty snack kids can make themselves!

Popcorn Balls

Melt marshmallows in a large bowl over low heat; add popped popcorn and mix until evenly coated. Scoop mixture into balls and let cool before serving.

Smoothie Popsicles

Blend favorite fruits (like strawberries and bananas) with plain yogurt; pour into popsicle molds or paper cups topped with sticks then freeze until solid!

Baked Sweet Potato Fries

Cut sweet potatoes into thin strips; toss with olive oil, salt, and pepper. Bake in a preheated oven at 425 degrees for 15-20 minutes.

Frozen Banana Bites

Slice ripe bananas into coins then freeze on a baking sheet lined with parchment paper until solid. Dip frozen banana coins in melted dark chocolate then place back onto the baking sheet to set before serving!

Zucchini Fritters

Mix grated zucchini, egg whites, and whole wheat flour to form small patties; pan fry until golden brown on each side in olive oil or butter substitute.

Cheese Quesadilla

Spread shredded cheese between two soft tortillas; heat in a skillet until the cheese is melted and the tortillas are crispy. Cut into triangles for easy snacking!

Baked Apple Chips

Slice apples into thin rounds; spread onto a baking sheet lined parchment paper then sprinkle with cinnamon-sugar mixture. Bake at 250 degrees for 1-2 hours, flipping chips halfway through cooking time.

Carrot Fries

Cut carrots into long strips; toss with olive oil, salt, and pepper then bake in preheated oven at 425 degrees for 20 minutes or until golden brown and tender.

No-Bake Granola Bars

Combine rolled oats, honey, peanut butter, and mini chocolate chips together; press mixture evenly onto an 8x8 inch pan. Before cutting into bars, refrigerate for one hour.

Veggie Dippers

Cut vegetables like carrots, celery, and cucumbers into sticks; serve with a side of hummus or ranch dressing as a dipping sauce!

Popcorn Trail Mix

Combine popped popcorn with unsalted nuts, seeds, and dried fruit then sprinkle with salt to taste!

Baked Sweet Potato Chips

Thinly slice sweet potatoes and spread onto a baking sheet lined parchment paper; season with olive oil, salt, and pepper then bake in preheated oven at 425 degrees until golden brown and crispy (about 20 minutes).

Apple Slice Pizzas

Spread peanut butter on apple slices; top with mini marshmallows and dark chocolate chips then microwave for 30 seconds.

Cucumber Boats

Cut cucumbers into thin slices, spread cream cheese onto each slice then layer with shredded carrots, chopped tomatoes, and sliced olives!

CHAPTER 9

Desserts and Beverages

Here are some Homemade Recipes for Dessert and Beverages:

Chocolate Chip Cookies

Ingredients:
- 2 cups all-purpose flour
- 1 teaspoon baking soda
- ½ teaspoon salt
- ¾ cup margarine, mellowed to room temperature
- ¾ cup granulated sugar
- ¾ cup packed light brown sugar
- 1 teaspoon vanilla extract
- 2 large eggs
- 2 cups semi-sweet chocolate chips

Instructions: Preheat oven to 375F. In a larger bowl, combine the salt, baking soda, and flour. Set aside. In the bowl of an electric mixer fitted with the paddle attachment (or using a hand mixer), beat the butter on medium speed until creamy - about 1 minute. Add the granulated sugar, brown sugar, and vanilla extract to the butter and mix until combined.

Take One at a time beat the eggs in until well combined. With the mixer on low speed, slowly add in the dry ingredients until just combined - do not overmix!

Fold in chocolate chips using a rubber spatula or wooden spoon. Drop dough by rounded tablespoons onto an ungreased baking sheet (or parchment paper-lined baking sheet). Until the rims are golden brown, bake for 8 to 10 minutes. Cool a little before moving to a wire rack to finish cooling. Enjoy!

Cupcakes

Ingredients:
- 2 cups all-purpose flour
- 1 teaspoon baking powder
- ½ teaspoon salt
- ½ cup softened butter at room temperature
- 1 cup granulated sugar
- 2 large eggs
- ¼ cup whole milk
- 1 teaspoon vanilla extract

Instructions: Preheat oven to 350F. Paper liners should be placed inside a 12-cup muffin tray and put aside. Consolidate the flour, baking powder, and salt in a medium blending bowl. In the bowl of an electric mixer fitted with the paddle attachment (or using a hand mixer), beat the butter on medium speed until creamy - about 1 minute.

Add the granulated sugar and beat on medium speed until light and fluffy - about 2 minutes. Take One at a time beat the eggs in until well combined. With the mixer on low speed, slowly add half of the dry ingredients to the butter mixture, followed by all of the milk and vanilla extracts. Do not overmix; simply combine thoroughly.

Add remaining dry ingredients and mix until just combined (mixture will be thick). Fill the muffin tin cups with the batter evenly. A toothpick put into the center of a cupcake should come out clean after baking it for 18 to 20 minutes. Cool completely before frosting with your favorite icing/frosting. Enjoy!

Rice Krispie Treats

Ingredients:
• 4 tablespoons butter
• 10 oz package of marshmallows (about 40 regular-sized marshmallows)
• 6 cups Rice Krispies cereal
• 1-2 teaspoons vanilla extract (optional)

Instructions: Grease a 9x13-inch baking dish and set aside. Butter should be melted over medium heat in a sizable pan. Once melted, add in the marshmallows and stir until completely melted. Remove from the heat and, if preferred, mix in vanilla essence.

Add in Rice Krispies cereal and mix until evenly coated with the melted marshmallow mixture. Transfer to a prepared baking dish and press down firmly using a greased spatula or the back of a spoon. Let cool before cutting into squares. Enjoy!

Brownies

Ingredients:
- 1 cup butter, melted
- 2 cups granulated sugar
- 4 large eggs
- 1 teaspoon vanilla extract
- ¾ cup cocoa powder
- ½ teaspoon salt
- 1 cup all-purpose flour

Instructions: Preheat oven to 350F. Grease and line a 9x13 inch baking dish with parchment paper and set aside. Melted butter and sugar should be whisked together until well incorporated in a medium bowl.

One at a time, whisk in the eggs until completely combined. Stir in the vanilla extract. In a separate bowl, mix the cocoa powder, salt, and flour until no lumps remain - do not overmix!

After adding the dry components to the wet ones, stir them just enough to combine them. Pour batter into the prepared baking dish and bake for 25-30 minutes or until a toothpick inserted into the center of the brownies comes out clean. Cool completely before cutting into squares. Enjoy!

Fruit Popsicles

Ingredients:
- 1 cup of your preferred fruit, either fresh or frozen
- ½ cup orange juice
- 2 tablespoons honey (or to taste)
- ¼ teaspoon ground cinnamon (optional)

Instructions: All components should be placed in a blender and blended until smooth. Pour mixture into popsicle molds and freeze for at least 4 hours before enjoying!

Vanilla Ice Cream

Ingredients:
- 2 cups heavy cream
- 1 cup whole milk
- ¾ cup granulated sugar
- 1 teaspoon vanilla extract
- pinch of salt

Instructions: In a medium bowl, whisk together the heavy cream, whole milk, sugar, and salt until combined. Stir in the vanilla extract. Pour the mixture into an ice cream maker and freeze according to the manufacturer's instructions (usually about 20-30 minutes). Serve immediately or transfer to a freezer-safe container and freeze for up to 3 months. Enjoy!

Banana Bread

Ingredients:
- 2 cups all-purpose flour
- 1 teaspoon baking soda
- ½ teaspoon salt
- ¼ cup room temperature butter
- ½ cup granulated sugar
- 2 large eggs
- 1 teaspoon vanilla extract
- Three ripe bananas, mashed (about one cup)

Instructions: Preheat oven to 350F. Grease a 9x5-inch loaf pan and keep it available. In a larger bowl, combine the salt, baking soda, and flour. Set aside. In the bowl of an electric mixer fitted with the paddle attachment (or using a hand mixer), beat the butter on medium speed until creamy - about 1 minute. Add the granulated sugar and beat on medium speed until light and fluffy - about 2 minutes.

Take One at a time, beat the eggs in until well combined. Add the vanilla extract and the mashed bananas after that. With the mixer on low speed, slowly add dry ingredients to wet ingredients and mix until just combined (mixture will be thick). Pour batter into prepared loaf pan and bake for 45-50 minutes or until a toothpick inserted into the center of banana bread comes out clean. Cool completely before slicing. Enjoy!

Milkshake

Ingredients:
• 2 scoops vanilla ice cream
• ¾ cup whole milk
• 1 tablespoon sugar (or to taste)
• ½ teaspoon vanilla extract (optional)
• Whipped cream and sprinkles, for fixing (optional)

Instructions: In a blender, consolidate all fixings and mix until smooth. Pour into glasses and top with whipped cream and sprinkles if desired. Enjoy!

Apple Crisp

Ingredients:
• 4 large apples, thinly chopped after being peeled
• ½ cup granulated sugar
• 2 teaspoons ground cinnamon
• ¼ teaspoon salt
• ½ cup all-purpose flour
• ½ cup rolled oats
• 1/3 cup butter, melted

Instructions: Preheat oven to 375F. Oil an 8x8-inch baking dish and put it away. n a medium bowl, combine the apple slices with the sugar, cinnamon, and salt. Mix until evenly coated. Move to a pre-arranged baking dish and spread it out equally.

In a separate bowl, mix the flour, oats, and melted butter until crumbly - do not overmix! Sprinkle the oat combination over the apples. Bake for 30-35 minutes or until golden brown and bubbly around the edges. Cool slightly before serving. Enjoy!

Lemon Bars

Ingredients:
- 1 ½ cups all-purpose flour
- ¼ teaspoon salt
- ½ cup margarine, mellowed to room temperature
- ¾ cup granulated sugar
- 2 large eggs
- 2 tablespoons freshly squeezed lemon juice
- 1 teaspoon grated lemon zest (optional)

Instructions: Preheat oven to 350F. Oil an 8x8-inch baking dish and put it away. Whisk together the flour and salt In a medium bowl. Set aside. In the bowl of an electric mixer fitted with the paddle attachment (or using a hand mixer), beat the butter on medium speed until creamy - about 1 minute.

Hot Fudge Sundae

Ingredients:
• ½ cup chocolate chips
• 2 tablespoons butter
• 1 tablespoon corn syrup
• ¼ teaspoon vanilla extract
• Whipped cream, sprinkles, and/or nuts (optional)

Instructions: In a small saucepan over low heat, melt the chocolate chips with the butter until smooth. Stir in the corn syrup and vanilla extract until combined. Serve warm over ice cream topped with whipped cream, sprinkles, and/or nuts if desired. Enjoy!

Cherry Cobbler

Ingredients:
• 2 cups frozen cherries
• ½ cup granulated sugar
• 1 teaspoon ground cinnamon
• ¼ teaspoon salt
• ½ cup all-purpose flour
• ½ cup rolled oats
• ¾ cup butter, melted

Instructions: Preheat oven to 375F. Oil a 8x8-inch baking dish and put it away. In a medium bowl, combine the cherries with the sugar, cinnamon, and salt. Mix until evenly coated. Move to a pre-arranged baking dish and spread it out equally.

In a separate bowl, mix the flour, oats, and melted butter until crumbly - do not overmix! Sprinkle the oat mixture over the top of cherries. Bake for 30-35 minutes or until golden brown and bubbly around the edges. Cool slightly before serving. Enjoy!

Coconut Macaroons

Ingredients:
- 3 cups sweetened shredded coconut
- ¾ cup granulated sugar
- 2 large egg whites
- 1 teaspoon vanilla extract
- pinch of salt

Instructions: Preheat oven to 350F. Line a baking sheet with baking paper and put it away. In a medium bowl, mix the coconut, sugar, egg whites, vanilla extract, and salt until combined. Drop dough by rounded tablespoons onto a baking sheet that has been prepared. Bake or heat for 15-18 minutes, or until the edges are golden brown. Cool completely before serving. Enjoy!

Strawberry Shortcake

Ingredients:
- 2 cups all-purpose flour
- 1 tablespoon baking powder
- ¼ teaspoon salt
- 6 tablespoons butter, cold and cubed
- ¾ cup plus two tablespoons heavy cream
- 4 cups sliced fresh strawberries
- ½ cup granulated sugar

Instructions: Preheat oven to 375F. Set aside an 8x8-inch baking dish that has been greased. In a medium mixing basin or bowl, mix the salt, baking powder, and flour. Add in the butter cubes and use your fingers or a pastry cutter to combine until the mixture resembles coarse crumbs.

Stir in the heavy cream until just combined - do not overmix! In the prepared baking dish, evenly distribute the batter. Top with fresh strawberries and sprinkle with sugar. Bake or heat for 25-30 minutes, or until the edges are golden brown. Cool slightly before serving. Enjoy!

Mint Chocolate Chip Cheesecake

Ingredients:
- ½ cup graham cracker crumbs
- 2 tablespoons butter, melted

- 16 oz cream cheese, softened
- ¾ cup granulated sugar
- 2 large eggs
- 1 teaspoon vanilla extract
- 1/3 cup semi-sweet chocolate chips
- ¼ teaspoon extract of peppermint (or to taste)

Instructions: Preheat oven to 350F. An 8-inch springform pan should be greased and placed aside. In a small bowl, mix the graham cracker crumbs with the melted butter until combined.

Press mixture into the prepared springform pan and bake for 10 minutes - do not overbake! In the bowl of an electric mixer fitted with the paddle attachment (or using a hand mixer), beat cream cheese on medium speed until creamy - about 1 minute.

Add in granulated sugar and beat until light and fluffy - about 2 minutes. Take One at a time beat the eggs in until well combined. Stir in vanilla extract, chocolate chips, and peppermint extract (if using).

Pour batter into the prepared crust and spread out evenly. Bake for 40-45 minutes or until the center is almost set but still slightly wobbly. Cool completely before slicing. Enjoy!

CHAPTER 10

Tips for Making Healthy Eating Fun for Kids

1. Allow them to help with meal planning and grocery shopping: Involve kids in the process by letting them pick out healthy recipes, or suggest new ingredients they'd like to try. Make a game of finding the healthiest items on your grocery list.

2. Get creative with food presentation: Create fun shapes and characters with vegetables and fruits for younger children, or make artful arrangements for older kids. Use toothpicks and other edible decorations to turn ordinary snacks into works of art!

3. Try themed meals: Choose a theme such as "pirates" or "dinosaurs" and create dishes that fit it—think dinosaur-shaped sandwiches or pirate-themed fruit platters!

4. Host a healthy cooking competition: Have each family member create a healthy dish and then let everyone vote on the winner!

5. Make it a game: See how many vegetables your kids can fit onto one plate or have them race to see who can eat their food the fastest (without making themselves sick!).

6. Let them experiment in the kitchen: Even young children can help out in small ways, such as mixing ingredients or adding toppings to snacks. This will make mealtime more fun for them and give you some extra help too!

7. Have a "taste test": Let your kids try different healthy foods and rate them on a scale of one to five stars. This will make it more fun for them to try new things!

8. Make it a family affair: Have everyone sit down together at the table to enjoy meals and snacks. This will foster healthy eating habits, while also giving you quality time with your children.

9. Offer rewards: Offer small rewards such as stickers or extra screen time for trying new healthy foods. This will motivate them to keep up their good habits!

10. Celebrate their accomplishments: Make sure to praise your kids for making healthy choices. This will encourage them to keep up the good work!

CONCLUSION

This book has provided a wealth of information and recipes to help kids fight cancer. By incorporating the healthy and nutritious cancer-fighting recipes in this book, kids can gain an advantage over their diagnosis by eating well and staying strong.

Not only will these recipes provide sustenance for their bodies, but they will also bring joy to the table with delicious flavors that everyone can enjoy. With this cookbook, parents have access to meals that are both convenient and nourishing for their child's health journey.

I hope that these recipes become staples in your kitchen as you continue on this challenging yet rewarding journey with your child.

Overall, this book provided valuable information on how to make cooking an enjoyable experience for kids and their families, even when faced with a cancer diagnosis. Recipes are not only nutritious but are also a fun way to share meals with children who are undergoing treatment.

Parents, caregivers, and children alike can now enjoy nutritious food that is packed with cancer-fighting nutrients and potentially reduce their risk of cancer-related complications in the future.

With clear instructions on how and why to eat for wellness, this book has the power to make a lasting impact on every reader's life. So take your cooking skills to the next level and share the joy of cooking with your children, one healthy and delicious meal at a time.

The fight against cancer is a long and arduous one, but by eating well, kids can gain an advantage. We hope that this cookbook has provided you with the tools to nourish your child's body as they battle cancer. With these recipes, we wish them strength and courage throughout their journey toward recovery.